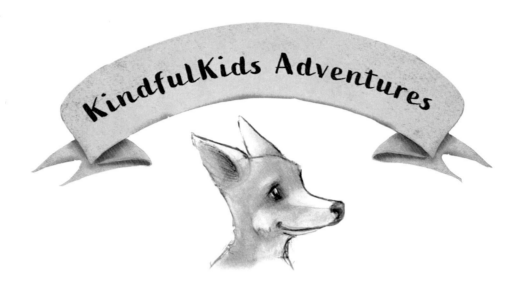

KindfulKids Adventures

The Quest for Kindness

A Fun and Interactive Path to Mindfulness

Written by Patricia Leitch

Illustrated by Soledad Cook

To Cotts and Rocky,

Your kind hearts are a gift and inspiration.

The Kindest Animal in the Forest
Copyright© 2018
Published by Level Above ™ Publishing in the United States of America.
For information go to kindfulkids.com

ISBN: 978-0-9980349-0-4

First Edition

Foreword

*D*anny the Dingo Dog sets out to teach kids more than just yoga as he embarks on a quest to find the kindest animal in the forest. His wise friend, Freddy, sends him into the Mystical Forest to meet lovable characters, practice yoga poses, and learn important lessons about kindness and mindfulness.

Designed for parents and others who care for children, this book introduces children to yoga and the deep breathing that accompanies it. Kids look at illustrations of yoga poses and hear details on how to practice them while experiencing Danny's adventures with his friends. No yoga knowledge is needed to enjoy this book aimed at cultivating children's natural capacities for authentic well-being.

Warning: This book may cause relaxation, calm and bring about a general feeling of joy.

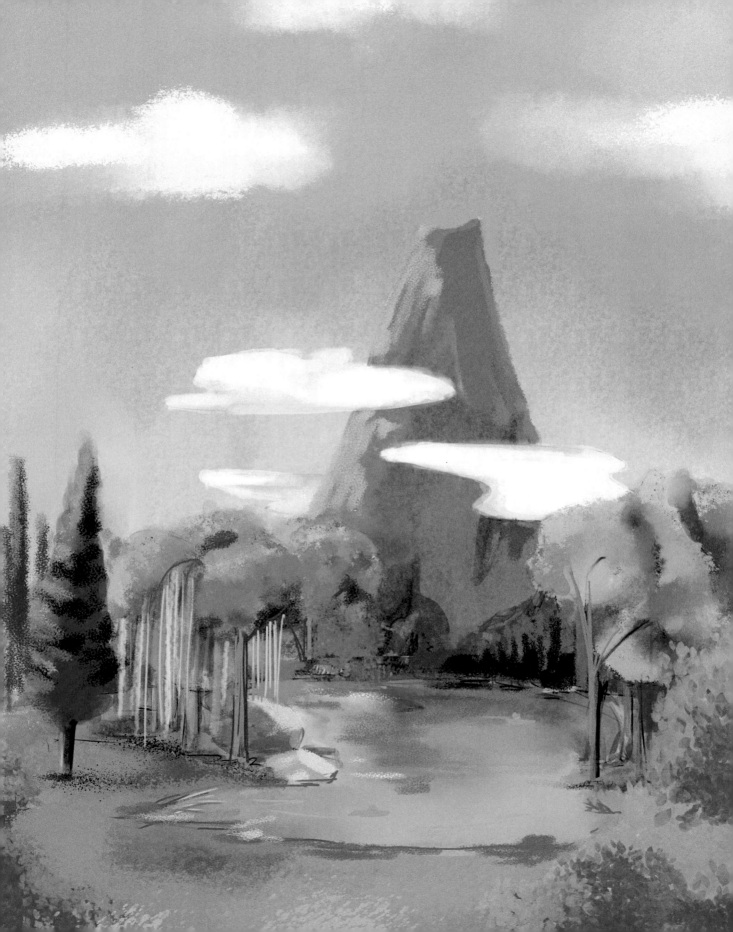

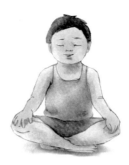

Welcome to KindfulKids Adventures

The KindfulKids Adventure Series takes children on an interactive journey aimed at bringing about a relaxed body and calm state of mind. No yoga or mindfulness experience is necessary to engage young learners' on adventures guided by adorable animal friends.

The stories are designed with illustrations on the left and narration on the right. Fold the book at the crease so the child may view the illustrations while the reader can recite the story and yoga pose instructions.

Read the book in a location where you can be face to face with the child with enough space for stretching. Perhaps have a blanket or pillow nearby for resting at the end. Comfort and quiet is important to get the full benefit.

For younger children, you may choose to leave out some of the detailed yoga instructions and allow the child to simply find their version of the pose. Remember, the most important part of the practice is full, deep breaths, not perfect poses.

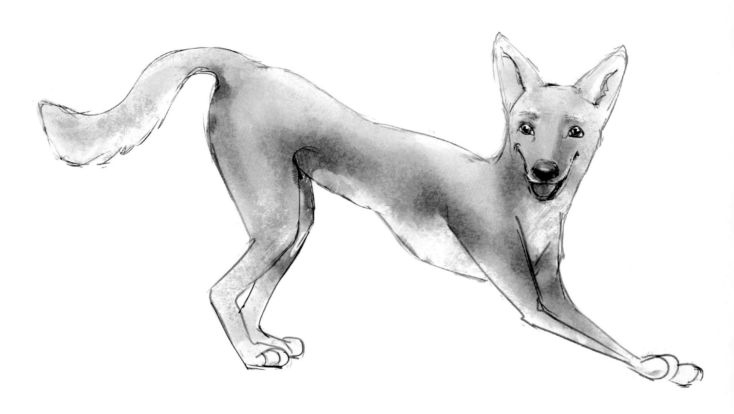

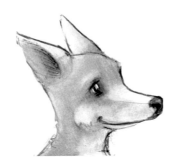

Hi kids. I'm Danny the Dingo dog. I have traveled a super long way from the Outback of Australia to find the kindest creature in the forest. Kindness means being nice to others without expecting anything in return. Who do you think is the kindest animal? And what makes them so kind?

To discover the answer, we need to practice yoga poses and breathe deep. Let's get started in my favorite pose.

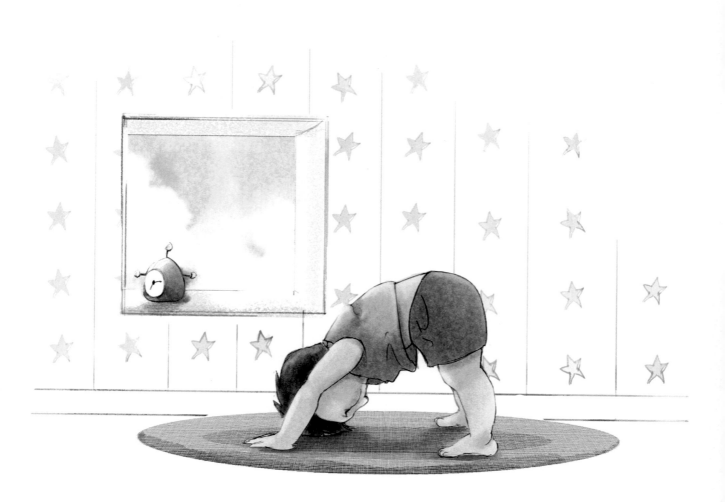

Danny's Downward Facing Dog Pose

Place your hands and feet flat on the floor. Move your hips up in the air. Bend your knees a bit. Relax your head. Push your heels into the ground and the most important part, breathe deep. I will count with you.

Inhale 1, 2, 3, 4 and 5
Exhale 1, 2, 3, 4, 5 and 6

Stay in the pose and try this breathing two more times.

When you are finished, bend your knees and sit down in a comfortable position.

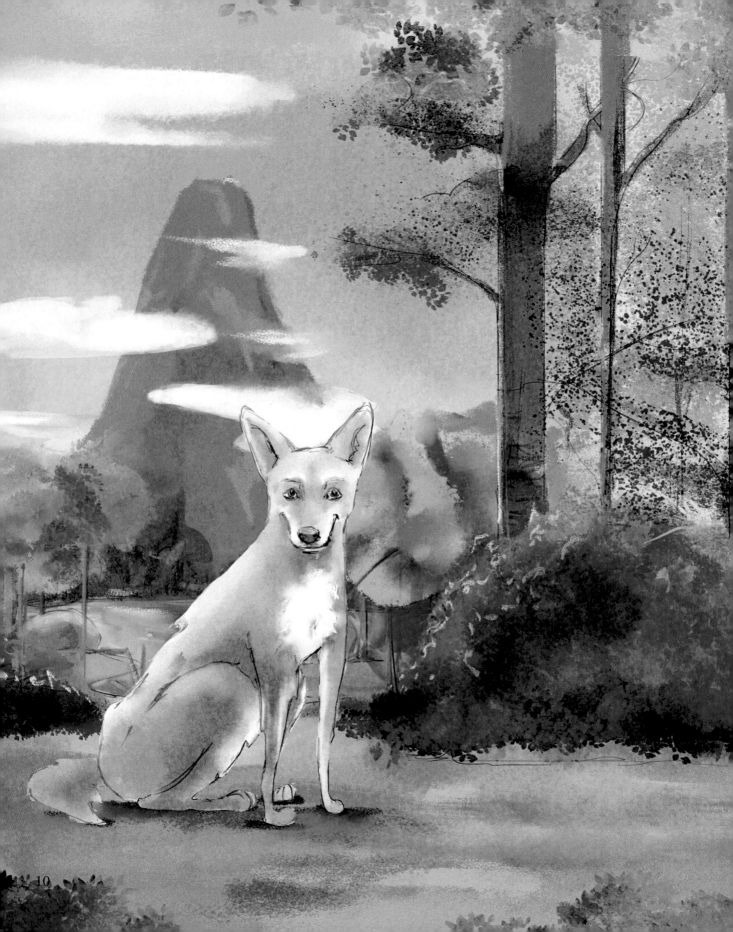

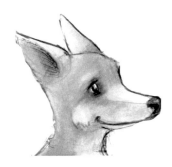

That stretch felt great. I'm excited to begin our journey. To find the kindest creature, let's do Limber Up Lunge Pose and head out into the forest to meet a very wise friend.

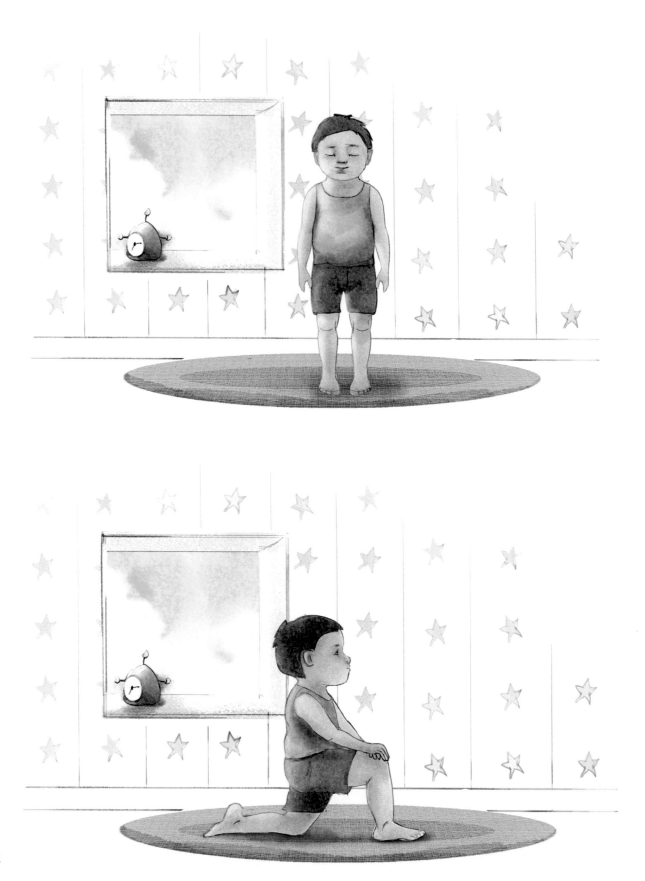

Limber Up Lunge Pose

From standing, bring one leg back. Place your back knee on the ground and both hands on your front knee. Then return to standing position. Do this again on the other leg.

The most important part of the pose is to breathe deep.

Breathe in and bring one leg back to lunge.
Breathe out and stand with feet together.

Breathe in and bring the other leg back to lunge.
Breathe out and stand with feet together.

Repeat three more times.

When you are finished, come to a comfortable seated position.

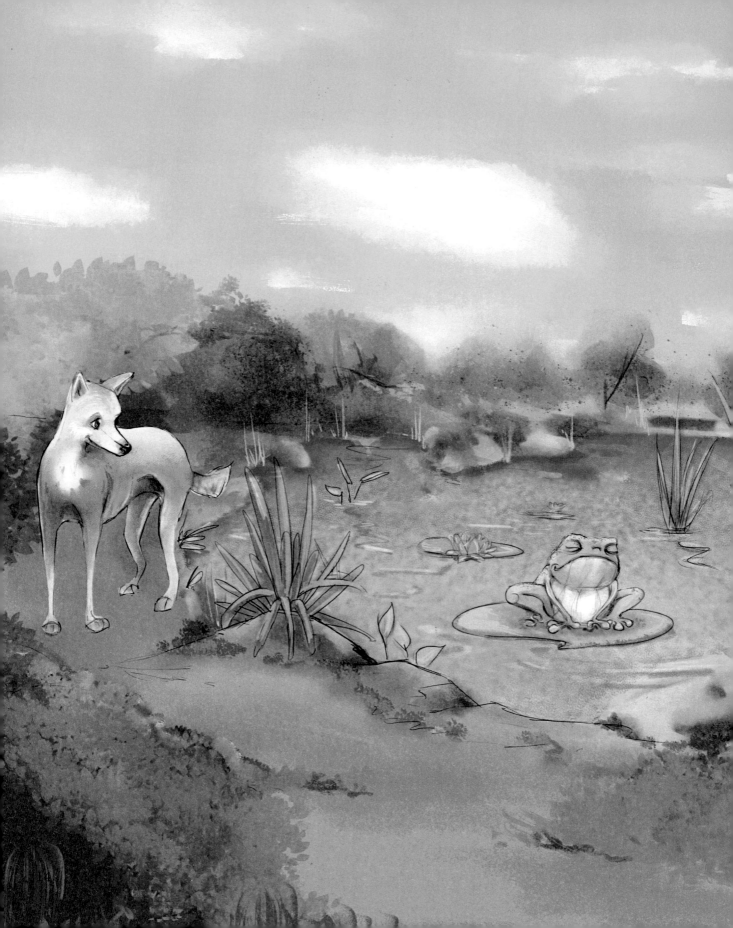

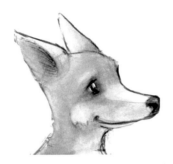

There he is! My friend, Freddie the Frog, the wisest creature I've ever met. Let's do Frog Pose, then ask Freddy what he knows about the kindest animal in the forest.

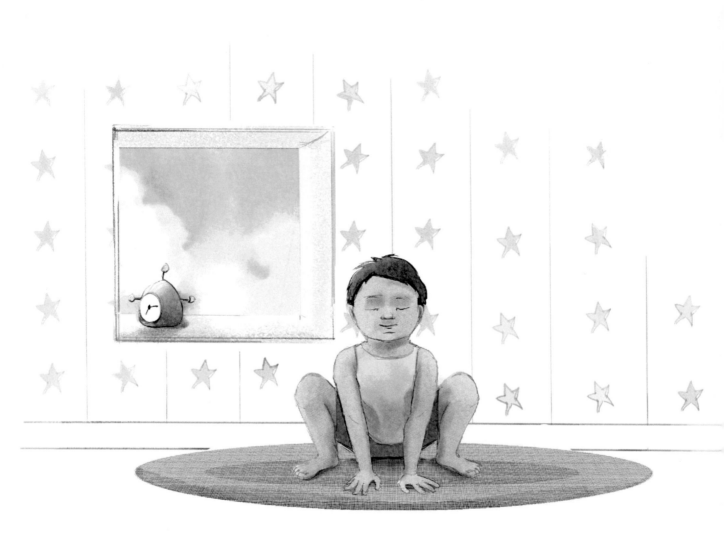

Freddy's Frog Pose

Stand with your feet a bit wider than your hips. Breathe out and bend your knees, placing your hands next to the inside of your feet. Stay very still and calm. Remember, breathe deep.
I will count with you.

Breathe in 1, 2, 3, 4, 5
Breathe out 1, 2, 3, 4, 5, 6

Stay in the pose and practice these breaths
two more times.

When you are finished, sit down in a comfortable position.

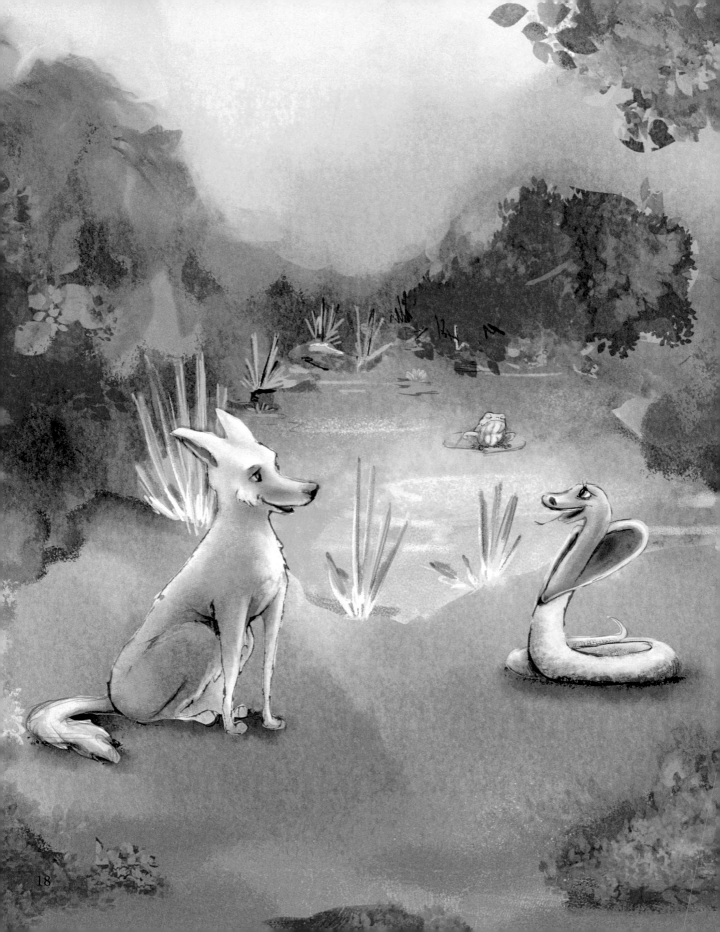

Good to see you Danny, I have been expecting you. To find the kindest animal, you must journey deep into the forest. I have asked Cathy the Cobra to guide you.

Hi Danny. I am Cathy the Cobra and this forest is my home. The best way to travel with me is to put your whole body on the earth, with your heart forward, like mine. We will slither through the forest together. When your heart is open, magical things happen.

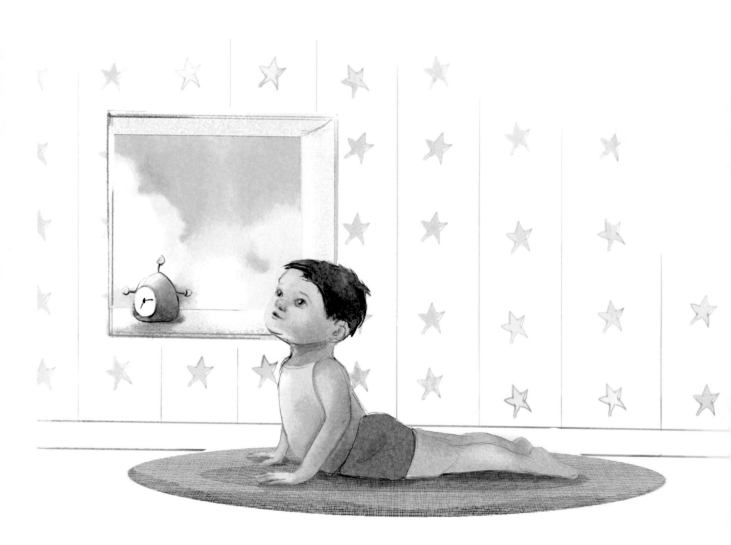

Cathy's Cobra Pose

Lay on your stomach. Place the palms of your hands next to your body on the floor. Bend your elbows. Lift your shoulders up to your ears, then relax them down, pushing your heart forward. Lift your hands up off the floor and breathe deep. I will count with you.

Breathe in 1, 2, 3, 4, 5
Breathe out fully, palms off the floor, heart open.

Stay in the pose and practice these breaths
two more times.

When you are finished, sit down in a comfortable position.

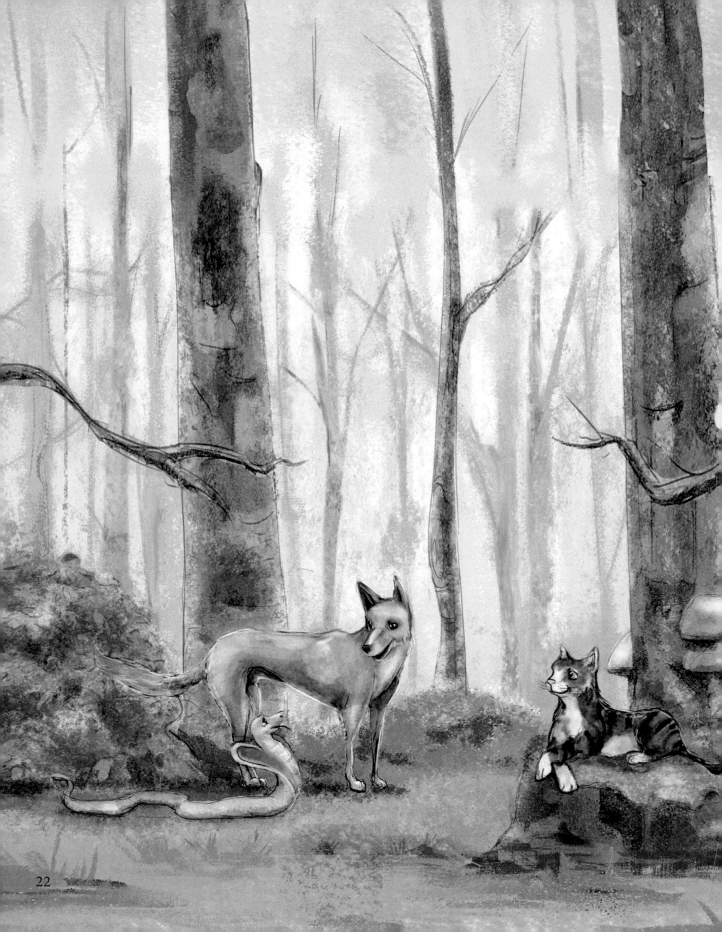

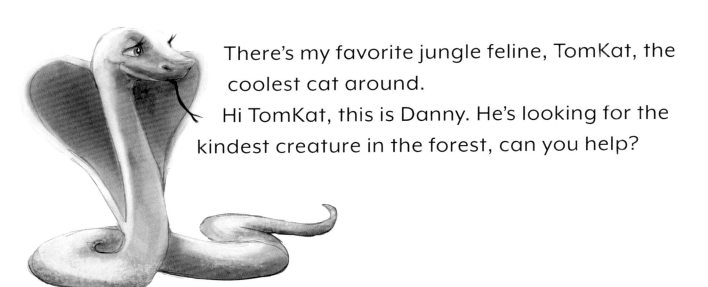

There's my favorite jungle feline, TomKat, the coolest cat around.

Hi TomKat, this is Danny. He's looking for the kindest creature in the forest, can you help?

I can certainly help you, Danny. Stretch and breathe with me first. You're going to need to be calm before your flight.

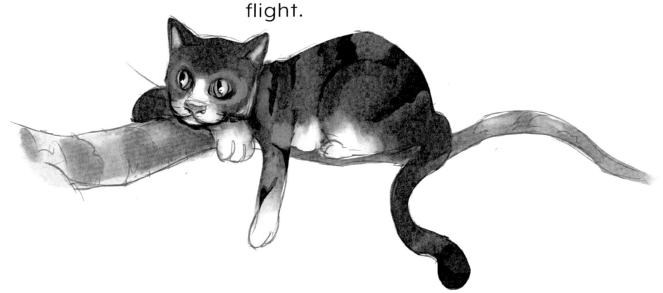

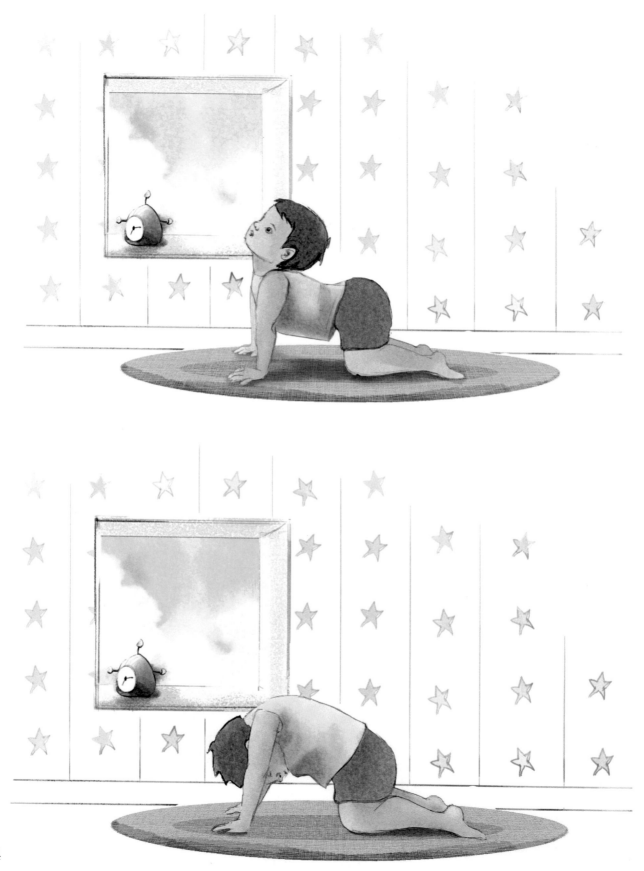

TomKat's Cool Cat Pose

Come onto your knees and place your hands flat on the floor, fingers forward. Inhale, arch your back and look up to the ceiling. Exhale, round your back, bring your chin to your chest and look at your belly button. Breathe deeply, I will count with you.

Inhale, look up 1, 2, 3, 4, 5
Exhale, look at your belly button 1, 2, 3, 4, 5, 6

Try this two more times.

When you are finished, return to a comfortable seated position.

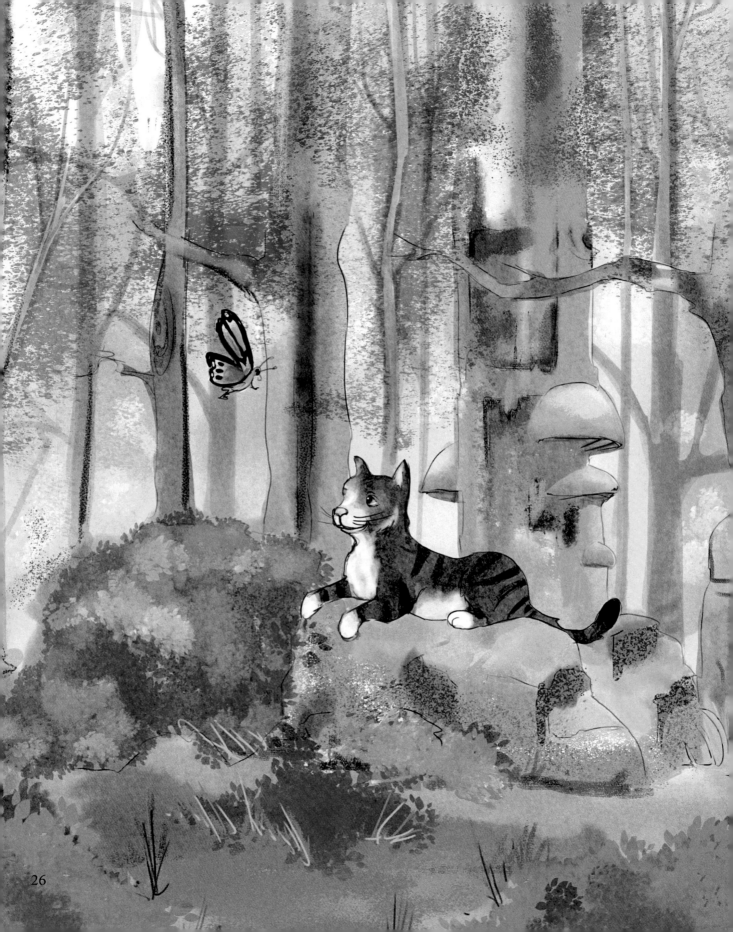

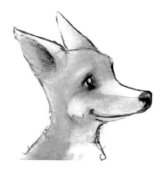

Flight? Another flight? I just got off an airplane from Australia.

There are no jets in this jungle. We have Blossom the Butterfly. She will help us. Enjoy the ride!

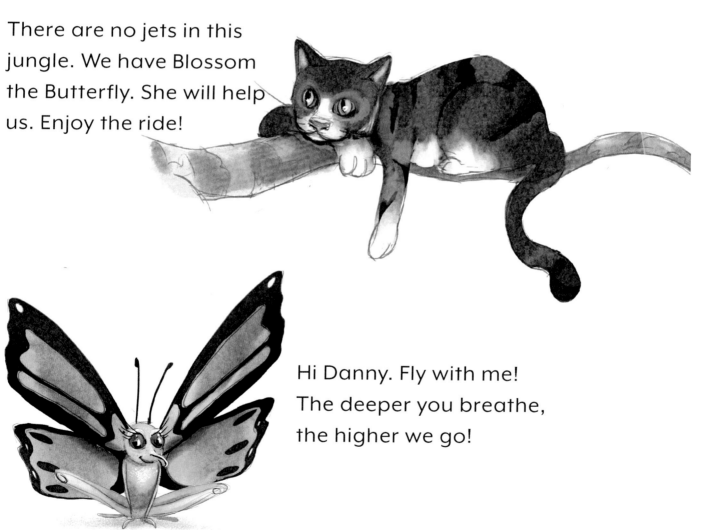

Hi Danny. Fly with me! The deeper you breathe, the higher we go!

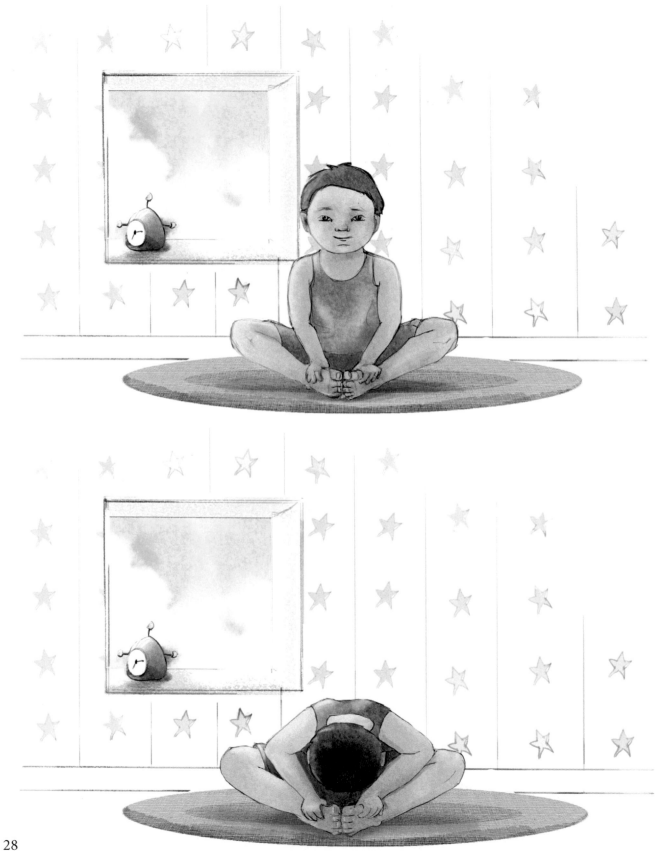

Blossom's Butterfly Pose

In a seated pose, bring the bottoms of your feet together with knees apart. Place your hands near your feet and breathe in deeply. When you exhale, bend over your feet, relaxing your head. Continue breathing deeply. I will count with you.

Inhale 1, 2, 3, 4, 5
Exhale 1, 2, 3, 4, 5, 6

Stay bent over your feet and breathe like this two more times.

When you are finished, return to a comfortable seated position.

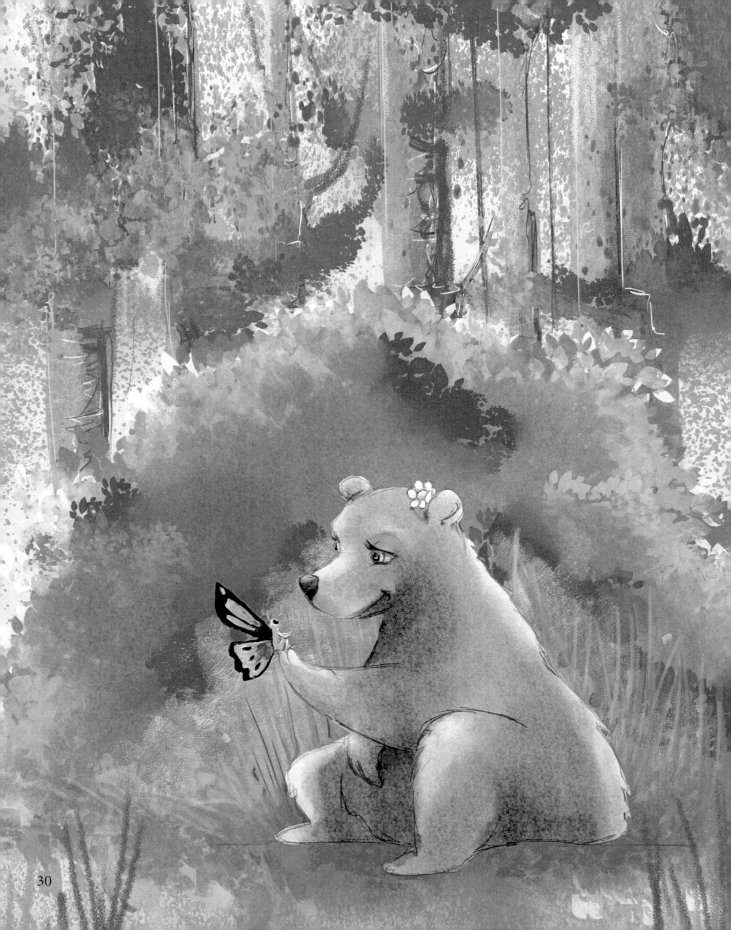

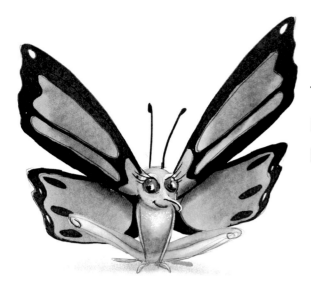

There she is. We found her. The kindest animal in the forest, Betty the Bear!

Nice to meet you Betty. We are here to discover your secret to being so kind. Can you share it?

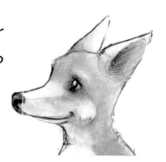

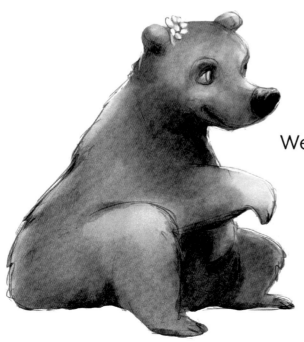

Well, it starts with a bear hug. Try it.

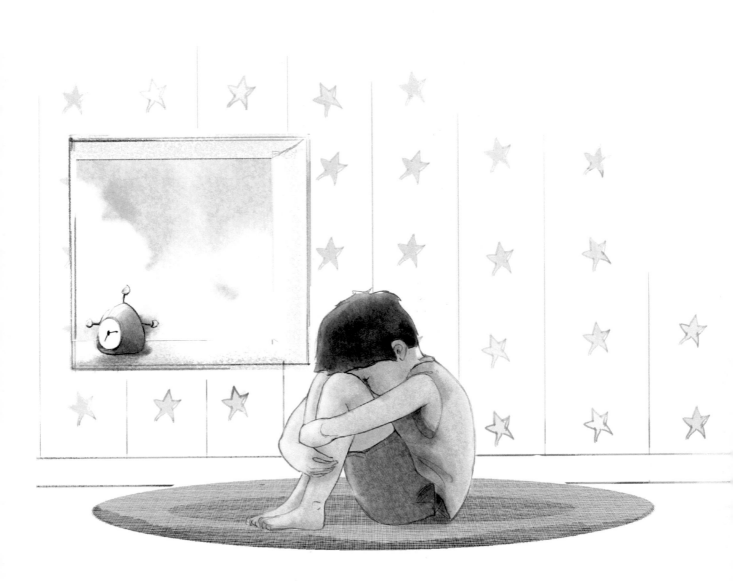

Betty's Bear Hug Pose

Sit down on the ground. Hug your knees and tuck your chin into your chest. Give yourself a nice relaxing hug and breathe deep. I will count with you.

Inhale 1, 2, 3, 4, 5
Exhale 1, 2, 3, 4, 5, 6

Stay in the pose and try this breathing two more times.
When you are finished, return to a comfortable seated position.

I am the kindest creature because I am first, kind to myself. Every morning I give myself a big bear hug, take three deep breaths, and say out loud, "I am a gift to the world and love myself for being exactly who I am."

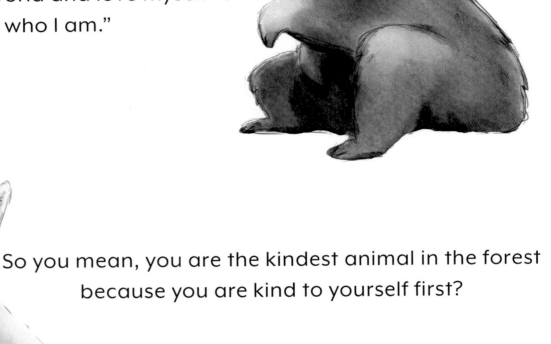

So you mean, you are the kindest animal in the forest because you are kind to yourself first?

Yes, exactly. When we are kind to ourselves, we can share it with others more easily. Loving yourself is where kindness begins. This is my secret.

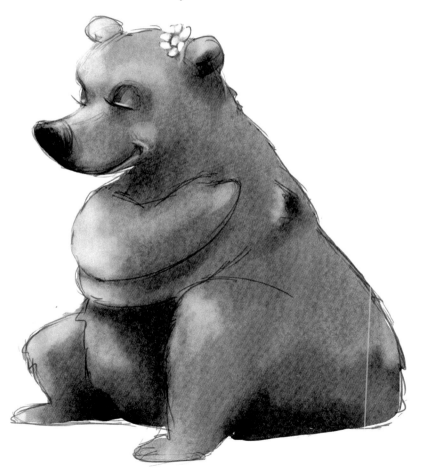

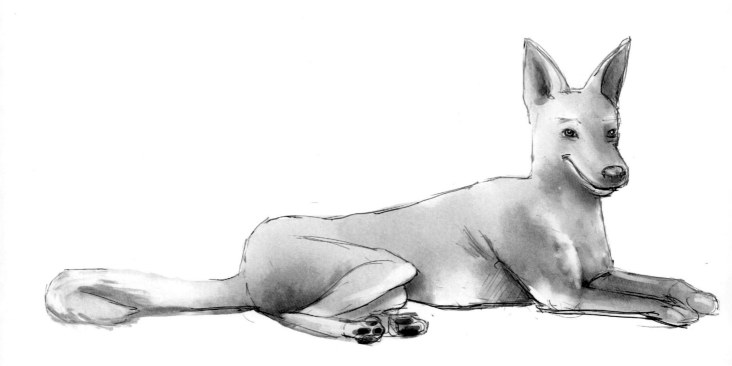

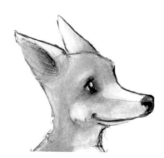

What great learnings from Betty. I never realized that kindness to others begins with kindness to yourself. Discovering new things always makes me happy. Let's do Happy Pose!

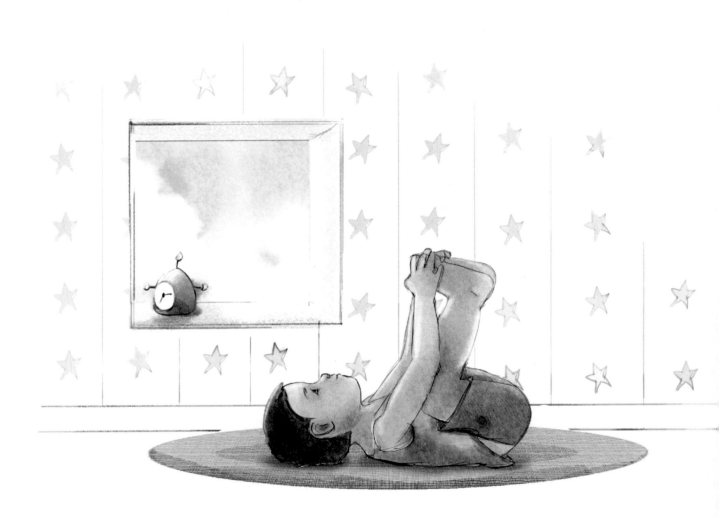

Happy Pose

Lay on your back with feet in the air. Hands hold the bottom of your
feet. Gently let the back
of your head rest on the ground and breathe deep.
I will count with you.

Inhale 1, 2, 3, 4, 5
Exhale 1, 2, 3, 4, 5, 6

Stay in this pose and practice these breaths
two more times.

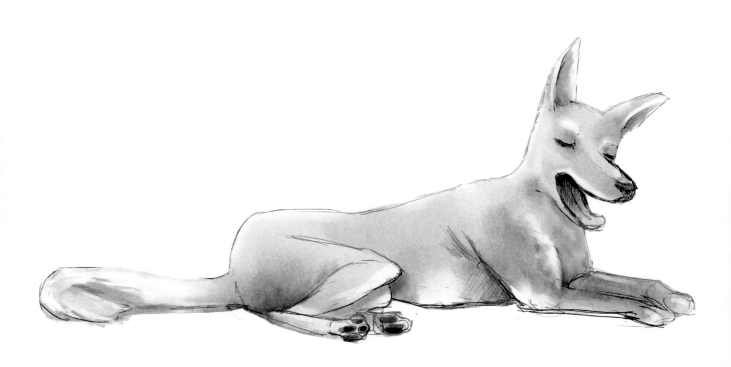

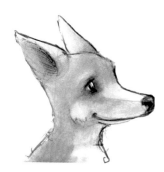

I feel super calm and peaceful. Do you?
Let's move into an awesome pose called "Relaxation."

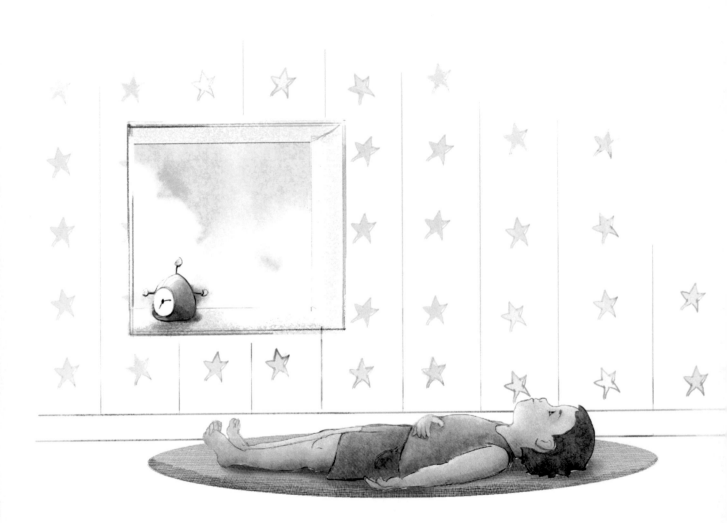

Relaxation Pose

Lay on your back someplace comfortable. Put one hand on your tummy and feel it move up and down as you breathe.

Feel calmness throughout your body and with each breath, just be who you are when you are still and silent.

Inhale, push your tummy up to the ceiling.

Hold your breath in and count 1, 2, 3, 4, 5

Exhale, let your tummy relax down.
Hold your breath out 1, 2, 3, 4, 5, 6

Keep your hand on your tummy and try this breathing
a few more times.

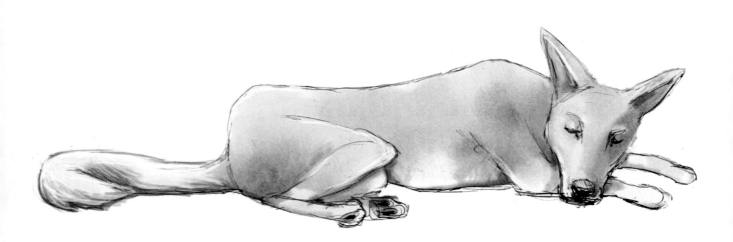

Yoga Poses

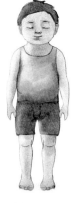

Mystical
Mountain

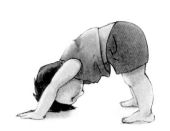

Danny's Downward Facing Dog

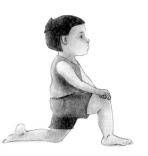

Limber Up Lunge

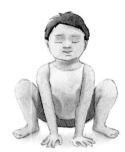

Freddy's Frog

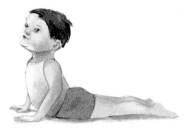

Cathy's Cobra

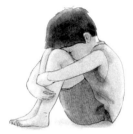

Betty's Bear Hug

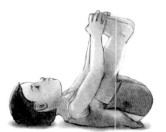

Happy Pose

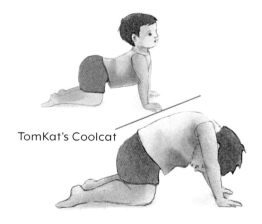

TomKat's Coolcat

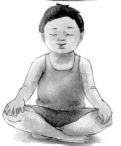

Blossom's Butterfly

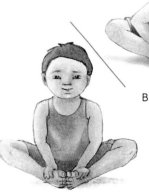

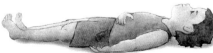

Relaxation

Reflection

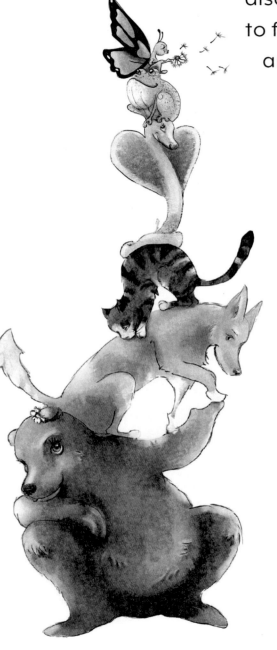

Yoga is a practice; there is no perfect pose. If you experience discomfort or pain, play around to find a version of the pose you are most comfortable with. Be kind to yourself.

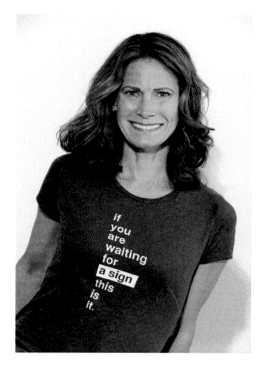

Patricia Leitch is an author and teacher who believes that early introduction to relaxation and mindfulness practices are critical for kids to succeed in today's media-fueled world. During her teaching years in the California public school system, Patricia realized young kids grasped social, emotional and mindfulness messages best when they were taught by lovable animal characters. Thus the creation of the KindfulKids Adventure Series featuring Danny the Dingo Dog, Freddy the Wise Frog and their journeys around the world.

Patricia is married and a mother of one human son, two dogs, four cats, and two turtles. Patricia leads yoga-based mindfulness classes in Palo Alto, CA and tells stories in schools and seminars around the country. For more information and to meet all the KindfulKids characters, go to kindfulkids.com.

Soledad Cook is a scientist and an illustrator who understands the importance of delivering complex messages through illustrations. She loves the art of storytelling and her illustrations are full of life. They are made with the sole purpose of taking the young reader to another world where they can meet characters and learn new things.

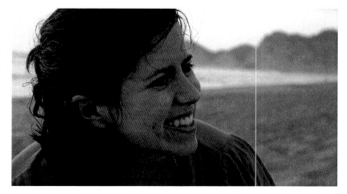

26660148R00029

Made in the USA
San Bernardino, CA
21 February 2019